# Intuitive Eating

# The Practical Guide to Develop Intuitive Eating

Jeremy Bradner

Copyright © 2020 Jeremy Bradner

All rights reserved.

ISBN-13: 979-8-6272-3151-8

© COPYRIGHT 2020 BY **JEREMY BRADNER** - ALL RIGHTS RESERVED.

The content contained within this book may not be reproduced, duplicated or transmitted without direct written permission from the author or the publisher.

Under no circumstances will any blame or legal responsibility be held against the publisher, or author, for any damages, reparation, or monetary loss due to the information contained within this book. Either directly or indirectly.

Legal Notice:
This book is copyright protected. This book is only for personal use. You cannot amend, distribute, sell, use, quote or paraphrase any part, or the content within this book, without the consent of the author or publisher.

Disclaimer Notice:
Please note the information contained within this document is for educational and entertainment purposes only. All effort has been executed to present accurate, up to date, and reliable, complete information. No warranties of any kind are declared or implied. Readers acknowledge that the author is not engaging in the rendering of legal, financial, medical or professional advice. The content within this book has been derived from various sources. Please consult a licensed professional before attempting any techniques outlined in this book.

By reading this book, the reader agrees that under no circumstances is the author responsible for any losses, direct or indirect, which are incurred as a result of the use of information contained within this document, including, but not limited to, — errors, omissions, or inaccuracies..

# CONTENTS

|   | Introduction: All About Intuitive Eating | 1 |
|---|---|---|
| 1 | Setting Your Health Goals | 5 |
| 2 | Understanding Your Body | 16 |
| 3 | Intuitive Eating vs Emotional Eating | 25 |
| 4 | Having The Right Mindset For Intuitive Eating | 35 |
| 5 | The 10 Principles of Intuitive Eating | 42 |
|   | Conclusion: Starting Your Intuitive Eating Journey | 51 |
|   | References | 53 |

Jeremy Bradner

# INTRODUCTION: ALL ABOUT INTUITIVE EATING

These days, diets are all the rage. It seems like more and more diets are emerging and they all have their own claims about how they will be the answer to your health problems. But if you have ever tried following any kind of diet, you would know that the effects and benefits of such diets aren't always sustainable. After some time, your body gets used to the diet and when this happens, you won't feel the benefits as much as you did in the past. If you're following a diet that is particularly restrictive, you might give up at some point because you miss the foods that you used to eat. Unfortunately, when you stop following these diets, all your health issues come back.

If you're stuck in such a situation, what should you do next?

If you're reading this book right now, it probably means that you're looking for a way to get yourself out of such a situation. You can do this by trying out something called intuitive eating. This isn't a new concept, but it is something that a lot of people aren't familiar with.

Intuitive eating isn't a diet. It's more of a way to approach food and health to make your life simpler and more fulfilling. Intuitive eating will help you learn how to tune into your natural body cues like feeling hungry, feeling full, and feeling satisfied. Through this unique approach, you will understand your body more and learn how to trust it, especially when it comes to food. By learning how to eat intuitively, you may get to say goodbye to diets forever.

The truth is, when we are born, we are all intuitive eaters. When a baby cries, their mother feeds them, and a baby will only keep on eating until they feel full. Then they would stop, go to sleep, and cry again when hungry. Babies rely on their instincts when eating and because of this, overeating is not really an issue. Even as infants grow into toddlers and young kids, they still continue to eat intuitively—only eating when they're hungry and stopping when they're full. For kids, there may be days when they eat so much food from morning until night but then barely eat anything the next day. More or less, though, kids will balance their food intake depending on their intuition.

But as children grow older, they start to follow certain rules and restrictions when it comes to eating food. It gets even worse when children grow into pre-teens and teens as they start giving in to peer pressure and they become more conscious about their bodies. Because of all these reasons, we tend to lose our natural tendency to eat intuitively. Instead, we learn:

- That we should finish all the food on our plates even if we feel full.

- That we should control our portions and restrict our intake so we don't gain weight.

- That we cannot have dessert unless we are good, thus, we treat it as a reward.

- That some foods are healthy while others aren't. And whenever we eat food that is considered bad, we feel guilty.

These are just some examples of the most common things we associate with food that make us lose our intuition when it comes to eating. The good news is that you can learn how to become an intuitive learner again and this is exactly what you will be learning within the pages of this eBook.

While intuitive eating is an innate tendency, the concept of using this approach to have a better relationship with food was created by Elyse Resch and Evelyn Tribole, a pair of registered dieticians back in 1995. Unlike the trendy diets that are taking over the world today, intuitive eating is an approach to food, wellness, and health without having to go through the challenges of dieting. When you look at intuitive eating from the perspective of a nutrition professional, it is all about focusing on your eating behaviors instead of focusing on rules and restrictions.

If you have tried different diets and you can't seem to find one that helps you reach your health goals or one that makes you truly happy, then you should definitely give intuitive eating a try. Through this approach, you might just find what you are looking for without having to feel negative about your journey.

As one who has re-learned how to eat intuitively, I can tell you that this approach has truly made a wonderful difference in my life. I myself had followed a number of diets but never stuck with any of them because they didn't really help me reach my own health goals. Although such diets may benefit some people, I wasn't one of them. If you don't feel like any diet is working the way you want it to, then you might be just like me and the many others who have begun their own intuitive eating journey. In this book, you will learn what intuitive eating is truly about and how you can start using this approach to build a healthy relationship with food.

From understanding your body better to learning how to adopt the right mindset for intuitive eating, I promise you that by the end of this book, you will have everything you need to awaken your innate ability to eat intuitively. When it comes to changing your life for the benefit of your health and well-being, there is no time like the present. It's time to learn why eating doesn't have to be a negative thing nor does it have to be a source of your stress. It's time to learn how to change your perspective and your eating habits so that you can finally achieve your body goals and health objectives. It's time to go back to being happy with your life because you neither restrict yourself from certain types of food nor do you have to follow strict dieting rules. It's time to take that all-important first step so let's begin!

# 1 SETTING YOUR HEALTH GOALS

We all have our own health goals and there are different ways for us to achieve those goals. If you don't have concrete health goals yet, this is the first thing you must do as you learn how to become an intuitive eater. Although there are certain steps you need to take to awaken your innate intuitiveness, the way you apply these steps will depend on your own situation.

For instance, if you are overweight, you would have radically different health goals compared to someone who is below their ideal weight. Since you have different goals, you will be taking different steps to achieve these goals. Another example is if you suffer from any kind of medical condition. You would have different goals than someone who is at the peak of their health and just wants to find a better approach to eating. In such a case, since you have an existing medical condition, you will have to be more careful as you work to become an intuitive eater.

In other words, setting your health goals will help define your journey. With these goals in mind, it becomes easier for you to determine what steps to take and what decisions to make for your health. Start thinking about your health goals now. If you're struggling with them, this chapter will help you out.

# How Can Intuitive Eating Benefit Your Life?

While setting health goals is important for your intuitive eating journey, you may want to learn more about this approach first, specifically how it can benefit your life. Intuitive eating enables you to learn how to tune into your body's natural signals. This is very different from dieting, where you try to control your body instead of listening to it. Also, intuitive eating doesn't involve lists of food that you should eat and food that you should avoid. Instead, you will learn how to become the best person you can be by making the best choices for your own body based on your intuition. Here are the other ways intuitive eating can benefit your life:

**1. It gives you more energy.**

Through intuitive eating, you will learn how to tune in to your body as you try to recognize your natural signals and how different types of food make you feel. This also helps you find out what types of food will give you the best effects. With this awareness, you can always choose the foods that make you feel great and which, in turn, provide you with consistent energy levels all day, every day. In other words, this approach to food gives you a better idea of the types of food that will help keep your energy levels up which can be very helpful in different situations.

**2. It will make you more aware of how food makes you feel.**

Intuitive learning helps you recognize how different types of food make you feel too. This happens because you are more in-tune with your body. This awareness helps you make better choices in terms of the food you eat. For instance, if you know that a certain type of food makes you feel lethargic, you may want to avoid eating that food when you know that you have a busy day ahead of you. The more aware you are, the more you can choose what to eat wisely.

**3. It makes you a more adventurous eater.**

As you learn how to eat intuitively, this can even make you more adventurous in terms of trying new foods or even new cuisines. This is an excellent benefit as it opens up your world to new possibilities. You might even feel more willing to try healthy foods that you never wanted to try in the past.

### 4. It makes food positive instead of being a "moral issue."

Intuitive eating helps eliminate the common "good" and "bad" labels attached to food. Instead of trying to restrict yourself from eating certain foods, you will allow yourself to eat whatever you want. This is an amazing benefit as it removes the guilty feelings you may have after eating foods that most people deem unhealthy. Also, since food is no longer a moral issue, it will no longer affect your mood. As long as you know that you are eating to nourish your body and make yourself healthy, then you know that you are making the right choices.

### 5. It helps you learn how to cope with your emotions and stress better.

A lot of people turn to food when they cannot manage their emotions and stress. This can be very unhealthy, especially if you lead a very stressful or emotion-filled life. But when you learn how to eat intuitively, you will also learn how to cope with these inevitable parts of life in different ways. This means that you can cope in a way that feels more supportive and beneficial to your life.

### 6. It makes you more confident.

When you no longer feel guilty for allowing yourself to eat, then you will soon become more confident too. This is especially important if you have issues with your body. When you learn how to become more intuitive, you will also learn how to understand and appreciate your body more. Insecurity will become a thing of the past as you find a new kind of confidence that will make you feel better and happier.

7. **It improves your relationship with food.**

It's important for us to have a healthy relationship with food. After all, we need food to survive. If you have been struggling with different types of diets, then your perception of food has probably become negative already. When you eat, you feel guilty but when you don't eat, you feel frustrated. Since you will be changing your eating habits and your mindset through intuitive eating, your relationship with food will improve as well. And the best part is, intuitive eating is more sustainable because it doesn't force you to follow rules. Instead, it allows you to find your own groove when it comes to your eating habits.

8. **It makes you feel more satisfied with your life.**

Finally, intuitive eating will give you an overall sense of satisfaction. As you feel all the other benefits of intuitive eating, you will come to realize that things are a lot easier in terms of your diet. You won't worry about what you're eating all the time and you can start enjoying the experience more fully. Since you will be in-tune with your body too, you will have a greater sense of unity between your physical self, your intellectual self, and even your spiritual self.

# What Are Body Goals?

We are currently living in an era where we are completely immersed in popular culture. Because of this, we are constantly bombarded with images of what the "ideal body" is, thus, we try to shape our bodies into what we believe is ideal. But should your body goals be the same as the goals of everyone else?

Sadly, if you focus on having the same body goals as the people you see on runways or in magazines, you might feel frustrated and dissatisfied with your body all the time. This is not the best way to live your life. Instead, the most important body goal you may try to have is learning how to embrace your body even though you're not completely happy with it. This is a lot more achievable and realistic compared to trying to have the "perfect" body but ruining yourself in the process. As part of your intuitive eating journey, your goal shouldn't just be about having the look that you desire but getting the desired feeling of looking good.

The body you have right now is the only body that you will have for the rest of your life. Therefore, when you're trying to think about your body goals, focus more on your own body, not the bodies of others. Try to learn how you can feel good about yourself even if your body isn't considered "ideal" or "perfect." If you can learn how to love your own body and feel comfortable in your own skin, then it becomes much easier for you to tune into your body to unlock your intuitive eating potential.

Body goals are the goals you set for your own body. For instance, if you're overweight or obese and you want to improve your health, then shedding a few pounds until you reach your ideal weight is a realistic and practical body goal. But if you are already at your ideal weight and you still want to shed more pounds to have the same body like the models you see in magazines, then you might start doing things that will affect your body adversely.

To become an intuitive eater, focus more on feeling happy and good about your own body. Come up with body goals that you know you can achieve. That way, you can be kinder to yourself as you work to achieve these goals. Take some time to reflect on your thoughts and feelings about your body then try to think of the body goals that you want to achieve. The more honest you are with yourself, the more you can think of realistic and achievable goals. Make a list of these goals and once you have finalized them, you can start working on your health objectives.

## What Are Health Objectives?

Once you have a list of body goals, it's now time to think about your health objectives. Health objectives are a lot like your body goals, but these also involve the steps to take to achieve them. To achieve your body goals and health objectives, you should always remember to take the right steps based on logical and ethical reasons. As an intuitive eater, you may want to focus more on your own habits, behaviors, thoughts, and choices. By doing this, you will learn how to become more intuitive, especially when it comes to your body and your health. Here are some tips to help you manage your health as an intuitive eater:

- **Think about your goals for proper nutrition**

Ultimately, your greatest health objective should be to learn how to "eat better." This may sound simple, but it does take a lot of time and effort to achieve. If you want to eat better to improve your health and your body, try to improve your nutrition too. Take a look at your current eating habits to give you a better idea of whether you are nourishing your body with the nutrients it needs or not. If you are, keep going! If not, you may want to make better choices without forcing yourself to change things drastically. It's better to take small steps towards proper nutrition instead of trying to make huge changes that will make you feel like you're on a diet again. Remember, it's all about using your intuition.

- **Make sure to include proper hydration throughout the day**

One of the most effective ways to ensure your health is to drink enough water each day. Drinking enough water provides your body with so many benefits. It also allows your body to adjust to your new eating habits as you move towards better health. If you're not used to drinking water, that's okay. Just try to make a conscious effort to swap out alcoholic, caffeinated or sugary drinks with this healthy beverage and you're sure to see the difference.

- **Eat regularly**

If you want to become a healthy, intuitive eater, eating regularly is key. To eat regularly, you may want to be more conscious of what your body is feeling. If you think it will help, keep a food journal or even a nutrition app to find out your own eating patterns. After a few days or weeks of tuning into your body and using these tools, you may come to discover these patterns that are uniquely yours. By learning these patterns, you can start creating a regular routine. This is a process that takes time, so you don't have to rush it.

- **Start with small portions**

While you don't have to strictly control your portions, it's a good idea to start with small portions whenever you eat. This allows you to eat everything on your plate without having to force yourself to finish what you have taken. If you still feel hungry after finishing the portion on your plate, then take another small portion. Keep doing this until you feel full. This is a great way to practice intuitive eating.

- **Focus on what you are eating**

Awakening your intuition takes time and practice. When you focus on what you're eating, you can also focus on what you are feeling. Try to focus on the taste, texture, and even the smell of each bite you put into your mouth. Try to focus on what the food makes you feel. More importantly, try to focus on whether you are still hungry, or you are already full. All of these things will hone your intuition.

- **Set goals for the different aspects of your health**

When you're thinking of your health objectives, consider your body, your mind, and your overall well-being. Therefore, you may want to include different kinds of goals and objectives such as:

    o **Physical health goals** like coming up with a new workout routine (more on this later) and practicing different breathing exercises.

    o **Emotional and mental health goals** like establishing a relaxing morning routine and learning how to meditate.

The goals and objectives you set for yourself would depend on your own needs and on what you want to improve in your life. Later, you can incorporate these goals into your plan for becoming an intuitive eater.

- **Get enough sleep each night**

Never underestimate the importance of a good night's sleep. When you sleep, your body gets the chance to repair and recover from everything you have gone through each day. No matter how busy your life is, make sure that you get enough sleep each night— this should be one of your health objectives.

These are some basic health objectives you can set for yourself. Some of these may apply to your own life while others won't. As with your body goals, take some time to reflect on what you want and what you need. Then you can come up with the best objectives to improve all aspects of your health.

# Tips for Setting Your Body Goals and Health Objectives

While intuitive eating is a lot easier than following strict diets, it still involves making a change to your current lifestyle. As we all know, making any kind of change can be a challenge, especially if the change is very different from what you are used to. But the key here is to make a plan, change your mindset, and take action. We will be discussing all of these steps in this eBook; we're just getting started! Now that you know what body goals and health objectives are, let's go through some tips for how you can set your own goals and objectives as part of your intuitive eating plan:

1. **Identify your ultimate body goal and health objective.**

When you write down body goals and health objectives, write down as many as you can think of. This is the perfect time to reflect on what you truly want in your life. Then put your lists together, analyze them, and try to determine your ultimate body goal and your ultimate health objective. For these, I am referring to the most significant, long-term change you want to achieve in your life. When coming up with these big goals, make sure that they are specific, realistic, and meaningful to you.

2. **Come up with goals and objectives that are uniquely yours.**

As you think of your goals and objectives, take yourself out of the norm. This is the best way for you to be more open, honest, and accepting of yourself which, in turn, enables you to come up with goals and objectives that are uniquely yours. For instance, if you are stuck thinking about what other people think, you might come up with a goal to lose enough weight to become runway-ready. But when you think of what you want, you might discover that you just want to feel happy and confident about your own body. For this, all you have to do is reach a healthy weight and maintain it. If you can step out of your comfort zone, you can self-reflect more effectively, thus, allowing you to think of what really matters to you, body- and health-wise.

**3. Commit yourself to achieving your goals and objectives.**

As you set your goals and objectives, you should also commit to them. Keep in mind that you are setting long-term goals, and this means that if you want to achieve them, you need to put in the time and the effort. For instance, intuitive eating is an approach to eating that will become a permanent part of your lifestyle if you want it to. Therefore, if this is your ultimate health objective—or at least one of your objectives—then you should commit yourself to it. The same thing goes for the other goals and objectives you set for yourself. Otherwise, if you don't commit, there is a very small likelihood that you will achieve the healthy life you want to have.

**4. Identify what motivates and inspires you.**

Most of the time, we start following diets because we are unconsciously driven by negative forces like issues with our body image, insecurities, fear or guilt. Unfortunately, if your goals depend on these negative things, you won't be able to sustain them for a long time. At some point, you will lose interest. This is probably why you find it difficult to follow diets for a long time. Instead, try to determine the things that motivate and inspire you. These positive things are much more powerful; thus, they can push you to keep going even when you are faced with challenges. Positivity is an important part of goal-setting as it will help ensure your success in the long-run.

**5. Approach your goals and objectives in a consistent way.**

No matter what your body goals and health objectives are, taking consistent steps towards achieving them will dramatically increase your chance of success. For instance, if you want to have a body that you're happy with and you want to become healthier too, intuitive eating can help you achieve both. This is an approach to eating that promotes consistency as it teaches you to listen to your body better instead of trying to change things that are beyond your control.

**6. After identifying your ultimate goal and objective, break these down into smaller, more achievable steps.**

Now that you have your ultimate goal and objective in mind and you have already done a lot of self-reflection, it's time to think of ways to move forward. To achieve your ultimate goal and objective, you can break them down into smaller, more achievable goals and objectives. These can also serve as the steps you take to reach your long-term "final destination". Trust me, each time you achieve one of these smaller goals and objectives, you will feel more motivated to keep going.

**7. Reward yourself when you reach milestones.**

Speaking of achieving goals and objectives, each time you do this, reward yourself for it. This is an excellent way to motivate and inspire yourself to keep going. For instance, if one of your smaller goals is to eat more fruits and vegetables, and you notice that you are now craving these healthy foods, then it means that you have successfully trained yourself to incorporate more fruits and veggies into your diet. Once you realize this, treat yourself to something nice like a movie, a spa day or anything else that will make you feel happy. No matter how small your goals and objectives are, if you achieve them, celebrate!

**8. Focus more on the process instead of the results.**

While you should focus on your goals and objectives—both short term and long term—these shouldn't be the only things you focus on. Reaching your ultimate goal and objective will take time. Even learning how to become an intuitive eater will take time. Therefore, you might as well enjoy the journey. When you focus on the process, you will learn so much more about yourself than when you only focus on the result. Try to learn how to be more aware of the present so you can feel more satisfied and fulfilled with your life. This can even help you in the planning process as you will look forward to the things you will do to achieve your goals and objectives.

### 9. Find support.

When setting your goals, try to think about your support system too. This might not seem significant in the beginning, but a support system becomes crucial when you are faced with challenges. Support groups, online communities, and the like are excellent places for you to find support. Also, it's great when you meet new people who are taking the same journey as you. Swapping stories and supporting each other will inspire you to keep going even if things seem difficult or hopeless.

When it comes to setting body goals and health objectives, the bottom line is to think of your own situation. Remember that everything you will do is for your own good. By now, you already know the benefits of intuitive eating along with a better understanding of what body goals and health objectives are. Just remember to use your intuition when setting goals and objectives and you're sure to come up with a plan to change your life for the better.

# 2 UNDERSTANDING YOUR BODY

Intuitive eating encourages you to learn more about your body so that you can start learning how to listen to it. In this chapter, we will cover all things physical that are related to intuitive eating. Eating is primarily physical. When you eat, you would use the different parts of your body. Even after eating a meal, your body continues working to break down the food for nutrients and fuel. If you feed your body with nutritious food, you can make it stronger and healthier. But it's more than that.

As an intuitive eater, you must learn how to properly care for your body to ensure that it keeps functioning optimally. To do this, the most important things you can do are to exercise regularly, learn how to control your urge to eat, and learn how to feel more love and positivity towards your body. By doing these things, you will come to understand your body better which, in turn, makes intuitive eating come more naturally.

## Establishing Your Exercise Routine

No matter what shape you have, it's important to keep yourself physically fit to stay healthy. If you already have your own exercise routine, good for you! But you can still learn a lot from this section because it's always a good idea to mix up your routine regularly to continue experiencing the benefits of regular exercise. But if exercise isn't part of your daily life, then you may want to establish your own exercise routine as part of your intuitive eating journey.

Even if you haven't tried exercising regularly in the past, it's never too late to start now. But if this is your first time to have an actual workout routine, then you may want to start slow. You can follow these tips to help you establish an exercise routine for yourself:

**1.    Plan for your exercise routine.**

For a lot of people who don't have exercise routines yet, this is probably because they keep making excuses not to engage in this physical activity. If you are one such person, it's time to put an end to your excuses. Exercise is an essential part of intuitive eating and health. But if you keep thinking that you can't have an exercise routine because you don't have time, you're too busy or for any other excuse, then you won't be able to start. Make a decision to build an exercise routine and make this part of your life. This is an important step towards your health and towards becoming an intuitive eater.

**2.    Think of when you want to set your exercise routine and plan for it.**

After making the decision to establish an exercise routine, the next thing you must do is think about when to do it. You can exercise early in the morning before the rest of your household wakes up. If you work from home, you can do it sometime in the middle of the day or in the afternoon. Or if you work all day, you can do it in the evening before having dinner. The time of your workout depends on your schedule and when you feel you can perform best. Your workout routine doesn't have to take too much time, especially when you're starting out.

**3.    Plan your exercise routine.**

The next thing to do is create a plan for your exercise routine. If this is your first time, then you should incorporate a lot of easy exercises like warm-ups, breathing, and stretching. Over time, you can start doing more difficult exercises to increase your endurance, make you stronger, and even motivate you to keep going. Typically, each of your exercise routines should last for about 20 to 30 minutes. But you can also shorten this to 15 minutes if you want, especially at the beginning. Just make sure to follow your exercise routine every day to really make it part of your daily life. Here are some of the most common types of exercises you may include in your routine:

- **Aerobic exercises**

These types of exercises are also known as endurance or cardio exercises and they're great for weight and fat-loss. These exercises will make your lungs and heart work harder, thus, increasing your breathing and heart rate temporarily. Some examples of aerobic exercises are swimming, biking, running, and walking.

- **Balance exercises**

As you grow older, your sense of balance may deteriorate. It's even worse when you suffer from any kind of medical condition. Unfortunately, when you have poor balance, this can lead to falls which, in turn, might cause injuries. Balance exercises can help avoid these issues so you may want to include them in your routine if you feel like this is something you should work on. Some examples of balance exercises are Pilates, tai chi, and yoga.

- **Flexibility exercises**

These types of exercises help reverse the tightening and shortening of muscles gently even as you age. Flexibility exercises are important since muscle fibers tend to grow stiffer and shorter as you age which, in turn, may cause pain, injuries, and even balance issues. Some examples of flexibility exercises are yoga and stretching.

- **Strength training**

These types of exercises are also known as resistance training and they typically involve the use of equipment like resistance bands, free weights, weight machines, and the like. Strength training is important for building muscle and preventing bone loss. It also helps improve your lean muscle mass to fat ratio. Some examples of strength training are weightlifting, pushing against walls, climbing, and more.

4.  **Start exercising!**

After you have created a solid plan for your workout routine, the last thing to do is to start exercising. If you're not a fan of exercise routines this can be quite challenging for you. When I started exercising, I only set a daily 15-minute routine. Now, I have increased my workout time to 30 minutes and I actually enjoy mixing up different types of exercises to keep my routine interesting and effective.

When it comes to exercise, the key is to keep motivating yourself. Even if you have a busy schedule, you had a tiring day at work or you just don't feel like it, try to stick with the schedule and routines that you have set for yourself. The more you do this, the more your exercise routine will become a permanent part of your day.

# Controlling Your Urge to Eat

Although you don't have to restrict yourself while eating intuitively, it's important to learn how to only eat as much as you need. Ideally, if you have learned intuitive eating, you will know when it's time to stop eating because you already feel full. Intuitive eating involves eating only when you are hungry and only eating until you have satisfied your hunger. This means that you should avoid overeating or bingeing as these can have adverse effects on your body. Before you learn how to control your urge to eat, you must first understand why you have a tendency to eat too much. Here are some of the most common reasons for this:

- When you are faced with difficult or emotionally charged situations, you cope by eating even if you're not hungry.

- You don't know the difference between the urge to eat and the feeling of hunger.

- You don't pay attention while you eat, thus, you don't notice when you feel full.

- You stock your kitchen or pantry with unhealthy snacks and food products that you cannot control bingeing on.

If you want to learn how to control your urge to eat and strengthen your intuition, there are steps you can take to achieve this. Try to make yourself more aware of your physical sensations and the natural signals of your body. The more aware you are, the more you will notice these things when they occur. Then when you get the urge to eat and you realize that you aren't really hungry, you can try the following:

**1.   Take a nap.**

Naturally, when you are sleeping, you won't give in to your urges. This is especially practical when you're sitting in front of the TV or just lounging on the couch. Usually, when you are bored, you get the urge to eat even though you aren't hungry. In such cases, try taking a nap. This is a great way to control your urge while resting your body too. Just don't nap for too long as you might find it difficult to fall asleep at night.

**2.   Try to relax.**

This tip is effective when you're feeling stressed. Stressful situations cause an increase in the level of cortisol (the stress hormone) in your body. When this happens, you will get the urge to eat with a special craving for sugary or fatty food. In such cases, try to find ways to relax. Find something else to do that you know makes you feel relaxed like drinking a cup of tea, playing games on your phone, taking a short jog, etc.

**3.   Learn how to manage your stress.**

Aside from learning how to relax, you should also learn how to manage your stress more effectively. Stress eating is a real thing and it can prevent you from becoming a true intuitive eater. Coping with stress can be very difficult for some people. If you are one such person, you may want to ask for help or support from those around you. But if you think that you can handle your stressors by doing other things, this would be very beneficial for you in the long run. Some ways to cope include meditation, practicing mindfulness, keeping a journal, or even meeting with friends and family to take your mind off the stressful situation you're in. When you feel better, then you can approach problems with a clearer mind and a different perspective.

### 4. Take a stroll around the neighborhood.

Another great way to control your urge to eat is by taking a stroll outside. When you do this, you would be distracting yourself with the scenery, the people, and even the animals that you see in your neighborhood. In particular, this tip is very effective in resisting the urge to eat sugary snacks, especially for overweight and obese people.

### 5. Brush your teeth.

I have found this tip to be extremely easy and effective. When you feel the urge to eat, you can either gargle with mouthwash or brush your teeth. This gives you a fresh and clean mouth that you wouldn't want to mess up by eating. Besides, foods taste weird right after you brush your teeth. So, this is another factor that can eliminate your urge to eat.

### 6. Make a fist.

This final tip may seem weird, but it might work for you. The explanation behind making a fist to get rid of your urge to eat is that when you tighten your muscles, this boosts your willpower too. Try it out! It might work for you.

These are some suggestions that have worked well for me. Some may work well for you too while others won't. You can even think of your own ways to control your urge. As long as the steps you take distract you from that urge, you can keep taking these steps so you can control yourself better.

# Learning How to Stay Positive About Your Body and Your Health

While intuitive eating is supposed to be a positive experience, it might make you feel more negative about yourself at some point. This is normal, especially if you have struggled with diets in the past because you want to change your body. While you learn how to become an intuitive eater, you may notice some good changes happening to your body. You might even move towards your body goals in the process. But if things don't change the way you expect them to right away, especially in terms of your body, try to stay positive.

Your body is more than just a vessel. It is your physical form that gives you the power to interact with the people around you, as well as your environment. So even if it's not what you consider "perfect," try to be more positive about it. Remember, it's the only body you will ever have! To make you feel more positive about your body and your health, here are a few tips to help you out:

**1.    Be kinder to your body.**

When you follow restrictive diets, you tend to place a lot of strain on your body. The same thing applies when you try following extremely intense workout routines. And you do these things to change the shape of your body into something more acceptable to you. But when you stress your body out too much, this will also cause a lot of stress on your mind and well-being. This will definitely make you feel negative about yourself in general.

Starting now, try to be kinder to your body. For one, accept your body for what it is right now even though it's not perfect. Then feed yourself with nourishing food whenever you feel hungry. Allow yourself to eat food that makes you feel good while you listen to your body, so you know when to stop eating (because you already feel full). Sleep, exercise, meditate, and perform other self-care practices to show your body kindness and make it healthier.

**2.    Keep telling yourself that you are beautiful.**

When you genuinely feel positive about your body, you will carry yourself with more confidence. A lot of people don't realize this, but beauty is actually a state of mind. If you feel that you are beautiful, then you will be beautiful. On the other hand, if you keep criticizing yourself or telling yourself that you have an ugly body, you will start believing these bad things. Try not to sabotage yourself. Keep telling yourself that you are beautiful, and you will become more positive about your body too.

### 3.     Practice mindful movement.

Mindful movement isn't the same as your regular exercise routine. When you practice mindful movement, you would learn how to tune into your body to find out what you truly feel and what you truly need. As the name implies, it involves moving mindfully to increase your awareness of your body, your thoughts, and even your surroundings. For instance, you can take a walk outside without a specific purpose in mind. As you walk, try to notice your surroundings.

Then make yourself more aware of your thoughts and how your body feels as you are walking. Do you feel your muscles ache as you take each step? Do you feel the breeze on your face? Do you feel the sunshine on your skin? Trying to observe all of these things teaches you to be more present at the moment which, in turn, makes you move mindfully. If you can keep practicing this, you will also be honing your intuition in the process.

### 4.     Surround yourself with happiness.

The best and most effective way to feel more positive about your body and health is by surrounding yourself with happiness. There are so many ways to do this and the more you expose yourself to happiness, the more inspired you will feel. For instance, if you have friends or family members who are very positive about life, spend time with them. You can also watch videos online about people who have learned how to accept their bodies and feel more confident in their skin despite not having "perfect" shapes and sizes. You can even think of your own positive mantra to say to yourself each day. Anything that will make you happier and add positivity to your life will help you out immensely.

Positivity won't come to you overnight, especially if you have spent so much time feeling negative about your body. Try to slow down so you can apply the tips I have shared along with other activities you can think of as you learn how to eat intuitively. First, learn how to understand your body more. Then take steps to make yourself healthier like establishing a realistic exercise routine and learning how to control your urge to eat. Take time to become positive and put in the effort to become more accepting. Trust me, all your time and effort will be worth it when you start reaping the fruits of your labor.

# 3 INTUITIVE EATING VS EMOTIONAL EATING

Intuitive eating involves relying on your intuition and your body's signals to know when to eat, what to eat, and when to stop. But there are times when you want to eat not because you're hungry, but because you are experiencing strong emotions. This is known as emotional eating and you should recognize this when it happens so that you can take the necessary steps to avoid it.

For a lot of people, it's a normal reaction to eat so that they can satisfy the emotional enjoyment or turmoil they are experiencing. If emotional eating really makes you feel better and you don't think that you can totally eliminate it from your life, then it's best to indulge in this activity in moderation. Also, when it comes to emotional eating, we often opt for decadent or luxurious food items so that they can help us get through the emotions we are dealing with. Sadly, emotional eating is very common, and a lot of people engage in it regularly.

Emotional eating occurs when any kind of emotion pushes you to start eating. Even eating because you're bored is considered a form of emotional eating. Often, though, emotional eating occurs even when you don't feel any physical hunger. Usually, emotional eating has a tendency to:

- Cause you to feel strong cravings that are seemingly insatiable.

- Come out of nowhere and persist even though you feel full.

- Make you feel ashamed, guilty or negative, especially when you give in.

One of the most dangerous things about emotional eating is that it can become a pattern which, in turn, may affect you in the long run. This is an issue that affects both men and women of all ages. Even children are prone to emotional eating, especially when parents use food to reward them for good behavior. If you have kids, be aware of this issue so your children don't grow up to be emotional eaters.

Emotional eating is a very powerful thing. Sometimes, you might even feel like you're physically hungry when you're actually just feeling intense emotions. When you give in to these emotions and start indulging in unhealthy food, this may lead to mindless eating. In some cases, you might even space out while eating and when your awareness comes back, you realize that you finished an entire pie, a whole bag of potato chips or even a whole chicken!

It's also important to note that the hunger you feel when you are emotional isn't coming from your stomach. Instead, this hunger is located in your head and it's causing you to lose focus on all other things—all you can think about is eating the foods that you are craving. All you can think about are the smells, tastes, and textures of the food you want to eat to satisfy your craving. However, there are also times when you won't feel satisfied even if you have indulged in emotional eating. Then you would continue eating until you feel uncomfortably full. Only then would you stop, but you might feel ashamed, guilty, and regretful after.

As you can see, this type of eating can create a harmful cycle that pushes you to feel negatively about food, about your body (especially if you gain weight), and about yourself. If you want to avoid giving into emotional eating, then you should know the common factors that contribute to it. These are:

- **Your physiology**

When you allow yourself to become too tired or too hungry, this may lead to emotional eating. Not caring for your body in the right way makes you vulnerable to the lure of your emotions. Then you won't have enough self-control to fight off your urges and cravings.

- **Food being your sole source of pleasure**

Although food should be your happy place, it shouldn't be your only source of pleasure or joy. In life, there are so many things that can bring you pleasure so if you want to break your emotional eating habit, try to find out what these things are for you. That way, you can deal with your emotions in different ways whether the emotions you feel are good or bad.

- **Not being aware of your actions**

This can cause you to give in to emotional eating and to continue eating even though you're already full. Unless you learn how to become more aware of your thoughts and actions, it will be very difficult for you to realize that emotional eating has already won as you have fallen victim to it yet again.

- **Having negative feelings about your body**

When you don't feel too great about your body, you won't care what you put into it. This is especially harmful when you feel negative emotions as you would give in to emotional eating and when you're done, you would feel even worse about yourself. This is one of the reasons why it's important to learn how to love and accept your body—so you won't do anything to abuse it.

- **Not knowing how to cope with intense emotions**

Finally, the most common factor that may contribute to emotional eating is not knowing how to cope with powerful emotions. When you feel these emotions, it's a lot easier for you to eat so you can feel better instead of trying to deal with your emotions appropriately. Don't worry, we will discuss this in more detail later on.

The emotions we feel can be either positive or negative. When the intensity of these emotions becomes unbearable, this is when emotional eating may kick in. Fortunately, there are things you can do to overcome this issue.

## Eating Out of Negative Emotions

It's very common to eat out of negative emotions like fear, sadness, anger, stress or even boredom. In fact, when you think about emotional eating, you would usually associate this with being unable to cope with negative emotions caused by conflicts, stress, financial or health issues, and fatigue. There are some people who may lose their appetite when they feel such emotions, but it's more common for these emotions to cause emotional eating. If you feel like you have a tendency to give in to your urges when you are experiencing intense negative emotions, you can use these tips to manage yourself better:

### *Accept the Emotions That You Are Feeling*

Negative emotions are part of life just as much as positive emotions. When you are faced with difficult situations, you would most likely experience these negative emotions as a response to them. Learn how to accept these emotions as they come instead of trying to deny them as doing this might intensify those emotions. Accept the emotions and allow yourself to feel them. Then you can move on to the next step.

### *Try to Find Different Ways to Cope With Your Emotions*

There are so many ways you can cope with negative emotions without turning to food. For instance, you can take a walk, read a book, take a day off from work, write in a journal, and so on. When it comes to dealing with specific emotions, I have found the following coping mechanisms to be very effective:

- When you're feeling angry, talk to someone about your situation, punch some of your pillows (or if you have a punching bag, this would be better), run outside until you sweat or write in a journal.

- When you're feeling anxious, try to meditate, join a yoga class, practice deep breathing, take a mindful stroll outside, listen to relaxing music or, if this emotion becomes unbearable, seek professional help.

- When you're feeling bored, try learning how to dance through online videos, do some research about something you're interested in, bake or cook something or plan a trip.

- When you're feeling depressed or sad, watch your favorite movie, don your most comfortable pajamas and have a good cry in your room, look for funny pictures and videos online, meditate or, if these emotions become unbearable, seek professional help.

- When you're feeling lonely, set a meeting with friends or family members, give someone close a call, spend some time in a restaurant or cafe to surround yourself with other people or volunteer at a local non-profit organization.

### *Learn How to Be More Mindful*

Finally, you can avoid emotional eating caused by negative emotions by learning how to be more aware or mindful of your actions. This takes a lot of conscious effort but practicing frequently will make mindfulness come naturally to you. When you're aware of your thoughts and actions, you can stop yourself from doing things that will affect you adversely—such as emotional eating.

## Eating Out of Positive Emotions

Emotional eating can also occur when we experience intense bouts of positive emotions. But the issue here is that you might think that it's alright to eat a lot in response to these emotions. For instance, if you attended a party celebrating a colleague's promotion, you may feel happy and excited for them. Even if you attend the party with a full stomach, you will agree to eat along with everyone else because it feels like the right thing to do. You might even make excuses for yourself to avoid feeling bad afterward.

Unfortunately, even if your emotional eating is caused by positive emotions, it is still emotional eating. Therefore, if you continue allowing yourself to eat whenever you feel happy, excited, and cheerful, you would still experience the adverse effects of emotional eating. It's okay to feel positive, in fact, I encourage you to. But when you have these intense positive emotions, here are some tips to help you avoid giving in to emotional eating:

- **Liberate yourself from food**

Food is a basic necessity in our lives, and we need it to survive. But this doesn't mean that you should indulge in food every time you feel happy. When it comes to expressing positive emotions, there are so many ways for you to do this. For instance, if you receive good news from your employer while at home, don't run to your refrigerator right away. Instead, play one of your favorite songs, turn up the music, and dance to your emotions. You can also sing your heart out if this makes you feel better. The point here is to find other things to focus on when you feel positive. Doing this will free you from your habit of always turning to food when you cannot find other ways to process your emotions.

- **Eat positively all the time**

Eating should always be a positive experience for you. This is an important aspect of intuitive eating. When you eat, savor your food, appreciate it, and feel grateful that the food you are eating will nourish your body and keep you healthy. If you always do this, it may help stop your belief that eating is a coping mechanism. Therefore, if you experience positive emotions, you will try to find activities that are "more special" because eating for you is already something good.

- **Allow yourself to indulge, but enjoy the moment**

Since intuitive eating shouldn't involve restriction, you may allow yourself to indulge when you are feeling insanely happy. Just make sure that you aren't eating mindlessly so you don't end up eating too much. Enjoy the moment, savor your food, and when you feel full, stop eating. By then, you should have already satisfied your craving while calming your emotions.

- **Learn other ways to cope with positive emotions**

In the same way you would find ways to cope with your negative emotions, you should also learn how to cope with positive emotions without resorting to food all the time. Some effective coping mechanisms are spending time outdoors, exercising, sleeping, writing, reading, spending time with others, dancing, singing, and even doing chores around the house.

# Learning How to Control Emotional Eating

Just as you can't learn intuitive eating overnight, learning how to break your emotional eating habit may take some time and effort. You should first learn how to control your urge to eat because of your emotions and then find ways to still deal with your emotions instead of ignoring them. It's not about restricting yourself. Instead, it's understanding what emotional eating is so you can change this habit into something better. Here are some tips for you:

1. **Know what triggers your emotional eating.**

While emotional eating comes suddenly, it is always caused by some sort of trigger. If you want to put a stop to this habit, you should know what your triggers are so that you can avoid them. Whether they are positive or negative, knowing your triggers is key. Here are some of the most common triggers that you might have:

- Boredom
- Childhood habits
- Feeling lonely or empty
- Overwhelming emotions
- Peer pressure
- Social or environmental influences
- Stress

It would be very helpful to make a list of your triggers to make them easily identifiable when you encounter them. If you can do this, avoiding the habit becomes much easier.

2. **Clean out your pantry.**

After identifying your triggers, you may want to start ridding your pantry or kitchen of the foods that you typically crave when you experience negative emotions, especially unhealthy foods. It's much easier to avoid emotional eating when you don't have food to indulge in at home. If you know that the foods you crave are just waiting for you in the pantry and you won't allow yourself to have them, you would feel restricted. By now, you already know that this feeling is counterproductive when you're trying to learn intuitive eating.

3. **Get rid of distractions that cause you to eat mindlessly.**

When you do allow yourself to give in to emotional eating, make sure to get rid of any distractions. You should be focused on what you are eating so that you can listen to your body and know when you have had enough. You can't do this when you're reading, watching TV or browsing through your phone while eating. Focus on your food and you won't have to deal with negative feelings after you eat.

4. **Get up and move!**

Exercising is an excellent way to release pent-up emotions, whether positive or negative. When you exercise, you are giving yourself something else to focus on instead of food. This works two ways because it prevents you from emotional eating and it also makes you healthier.

5. **Practice positive self-talk.**

This tip is especially helpful when dealing with negative emotions. Before you dive into your usual unhealthy coping mechanisms like emotional eating, try to practice positive self-talk first. Talk about your situation, your feelings, and how you can make things better. If possible, try to find the silver lining to ease the stress and negativity you feel. Hopefully, after your positive self-talk, you won't have the urge to raid your refrigerator anymore.

## 6. Learn how to say "no" to yourself.

Intuitive eating teaches you to be kinder to yourself. However, this doesn't mean that you should give in to all of your urges. You must learn how to determine whether the things you want will benefit you or cause you harm. If it's the latter, learn how to say "no" to yourself. This may take some conscious effort on your part, but it will surely benefit your life in the long run.

## 7. Learn different coping skills.

Finally, try to learn different coping skills when faced with powerful emotions. Coping skills differ from coping mechanisms as the latter are the activities that you can do while the former are the things you need to do those activities. Generally, coping skills can be classified as:

- **Taking action** like exercising, crying or doing chores.

- **Connecting** like calling your parents, setting a date with your friends or talking to someone about your problems.

- **Finding pleasure** like having a spa day, indulging in a glass of wine or buying something that you really want.

- **Soothing** like reading your favorite book, listening to calming music or getting a massage.

Intuitive eating and emotional eating are two different things. When you eat emotionally, you tend to lose control because you are too focused on your emotions. But when you eat intuitively, you learn how to control yourself by listening to the natural signals of your body. Throughout this chapter, you have learned a lot of skills and strategies to help you break free of emotional eating so that you can focus more on intuitive eating. Learning these skills will enable you to think of appropriate coping mechanisms for different situations. If you can do this (and all the other tips I have shared), emotional eating can be something that you have overcome during your intuitive eating journey.

# 4 HAVING THE RIGHT MINDSET FOR INTUITIVE EATING

Did you know that your mind is truly a powerful thing?

By changing your mindset, you can make it easier for yourself to learn how to become an intuitive eater. Aside from tuning in to your body and learning how to listen to your natural body signals, you should also have the right mentality to approach food and eating intuitively. For instance, if you always remind yourself to only eat when you're hungry, you will learn how to be more aware of your hunger. Of course, you should also allow yourself to eat if you want to experience the joy of eating as long as you aren't feeling full.

To change your mindset and become an intuitive eater, you must understand yourself better. Accept that intuitive eating isn't your current approach, but you can always develop and improve yourself to learn how to eat intuitively. Also, try to help yourself understand that intuitive eating is a habit that you can manage. Over time, it becomes a natural part of your life. When this happens, you may also discover that you have gained more self-control in terms of your eating habits. You won't have to worry about eating too much or losing control in any other way because your intuition is always there to guide you. When you notice this, then you know that you have truly transitioned into becoming an intuitive eater.

# The Importance of Having the Right Mindset

Right now, you might not have the right mindset to tackle intuitive eating just yet. That's okay. The fact that you're reading this eBook (and that you have come this far) already says a lot about your willingness to learn. Now, all you need is a nudge in the right direction and a few good reasons to change your mindset for your own benefit. To help you realize the importance of having the right mindset, here are a few reasons to consider:

**1. It helps improve your overall wellness.**

With the right mindset, you can approach intuitive eating in a more positive way. No matter what change you are trying to make in your life, adopting the right mindset will make things easier. In the case of intuitive eating, if you can successfully change your mindset to become more intuitive, then this will help improve your overall health and well-being. Your physical health will improve along with your mental and spiritual health as you become a more positive and accepting person, especially to yourself.

**2. It helps you achieve your body goals and health objectives.**

After setting your goals, creating your plan, and learning more about your body, another important step to take is to change your mindset. When you have the right mindset, you will approach intuitive eating from a different perspective. You will accept your current habits, let go of your past beliefs (especially in terms of dieting), and start working towards your goals. When you set your mind towards your goals, you will always have the motivation to keep going. And when you start seeing positive changes in your health and wellness, you will feel even more positive about your journey.

**3. It helps you manage stress more effectively.**

Stress is a great hindrance in life no matter what goals you set for yourself. When you are stressed, this affects your mind and body. If you allow it to, it will decrease your chances of achieving your goals, one of which, in this case, is to become an intuitive eater. But you can turn things around for yourself if you can change your mindset. With the right mindset, you can face any challenge. Since stress is one of the most common challenges out there, having the right mindset will enable you to manage your stress more effectively.

## Maintaining a Positive Mindset

Now that you know how important a positive mindset is, you should work on maintaining this type of mindset as you apply intuitive eating to your life. The good news is that there are many things you can do to achieve this. With practice, your positive mindset will become your ally.

### *Start Each Day With Positivity*

You can start practicing positivity the moment you open your eyes each morning. When you wake up, smile and fill your mind with happy thoughts. If you have plans for the day, tell yourself that these plans will succeed as you will give them your best. Say a short prayer of gratitude and appreciation so your day begins with positive things. Starting your day this way encourages you to maintain this kind of mindset from morning until night. Make this a habit so that you will always make an effort to be positive no matter what has happened the day before.

### *Focus on Good Things No Matter How Small*

To maintain a positive mindset, you should look for things that encourage it. Focus on everything good that happens to you no matter how small or insignificant these things may seem. For instance, if you have kids and they all woke up in the morning without a fuss, this can be something to appreciate. Or if one of your colleagues brought you a cup of coffee at work, this is another thing to be thankful for. By focusing on these things, you will train your mind to always look for the silver lining no matter how bad things might get.

## Use Positivity to Care for Your Health

Having a positive mindset can do wonders for your health. And if you want to maintain this type of mindset, keep working on it. Here are some ways you can practice positivity for the benefit of your health:

- Find activities that you enjoy to help you unwind when things get stressful.

- Find ways to make boring activities more fun and interesting.

- Maintain a journal where you write down all of your positive thoughts and experiences.

- When you achieve something, give yourself credit for it.

- Spend time with the people you love so that they can support you and make you feel happier about your life.

Simple as these things may be, they will all contribute to your positive mindset and to your overall health and well-being.

## Practice Positive Language

The things that you say always come from your mind. Another way to strengthen your positive mindset is by practicing the use of positive language. Whether you are talking to yourself or talking to other people, using such language makes things easier for you. For instance, when you keep reminding yourself that you can learn how to become an intuitive eater, then you will keep trying to achieve this goal. This is why positive self-talk is crucial, especially when it comes to breaking your bad habits.

## When Negative Thoughts Come Knocking, Stop Them in Their Tracks

Negative thoughts will always exist, but this doesn't mean that you have to surrender to them. Being mindful will benefit you when applying this tip as you will recognize negative thoughts when they come knocking. As soon as these thoughts come, stop them in their tracks before they can do harm to the positive mindset you have been building for yourself.

### *Learn How to Be Grateful*

Finally, learn how to live with gratitude as this is a powerful force that will help you maintain a positive mindset throughout and beyond your intuitive eating journey. Once you have strengthened your positive mindset, you can achieve anything!

## Approaching Intuitive Eating With the Right Mindset

Your positive mindset will greatly increase your chances of learning how to become an intuitive eater. Now, you can go back to the plans you have made and try to see how you can approach intuitive eating with the right mindset. For this, you would have to make sure that your approach to eating always has a reason or a purpose behind it. This means that you would only eat because you are hungry, because you want to enjoy something you have been craving, because you are celebrating something, or for any valid reason.

As long as you have a reason behind wanting to eat and your intuition is encouraging you to eat, allow yourself to. But if you just want to eat something to cope with stress, deal with your emotions or just for the sake of eating, then you may want to think of something else to do. This is where your intuition and the power of your mind should come into play. Here are some helpful ways for you to approach eating intuitively and with the right mindset:

• Although you may eat what you want based on your intuition, consider your nutrition too. You may want to remember that nutritious foods will make your body feel better in ways that unhealthy foods cannot.

• Consider learning how to prepare your own meals at home.

This makes it easier for you to choose exactly what you want to eat and prepare your meals exactly how you want them to be prepared. Also, planning your meals allows you to think about food in a more positive way.

- Keep reminding yourself of your goals so that all of the decisions you make will get you closer to achieving those goals.

- Always pay attention to your body so that you will only eat when you're hungry (or for any other good reason) and you will stop eating once you're full.

- When eating foods that aren't considered healthy, practice moderation. Learn how to find the right balance between pleasure and indulgence. Also, try to eat until you feel comfortable and satisfied, not until you feel too full.

- Open your mind to the possibility of eating a wide range of foods, not just your favorites. This will make things more interesting for you which, in turn, will continue strengthening your intuition and motivation.

## The Power of Your Mind

Your mind is truly a powerful thing. It is the final piece you need to complete your preparations for becoming an intuitive eater. By strengthening your mind, you can practice self-control. You can also consider your mind as the key ingredient that will govern your intuitive approach to eating. Now that you know how powerful your mind is, keep using it.

Empowering yourself by strengthening your mind and cultivating a positive mindset will help you unlock your potential for self-control. As you may come to discover, controlling your actions in terms of food (and even other aspects of your life) becomes easier when you have the right mindset. For instance, if you are stuck in a very stressful situation and your go-to solution in the past was to eat until you felt better, having the right mindset will help you control your urge. After you have learned that emotional eating isn't the best solution to stress, you can think of productive ways to deal with your situation and the emotions that come with it. Having the right mindset awakens your intuition and awareness—two things that enable you to take control over your decisions better.

By applying everything you have learned in this chapter, you can strengthen your mindset and create your own guidelines for intuitive eating. Use your mind to train your body until intuitive eating becomes your natural approach to eating. Over time, I can tell you that intuitive eating gets easier. As long as you keep practicing and you apply all of the tips and guidelines you have learned, you will soon awaken your intuition and learn how to eat by following it. You may find it new and challenging in the beginning but if you keep with it, intuitive eating will become your way of life.

# 5 THE 10 PRINCIPLES OF INTUITIVE EATING

For this final chapter, I will share with you the 10 principles of intuitive eating. It's important to understand these principles as they will also serve as your guide for when you try to become a more intuitive eater. With everything you have learned in the past four chapters, you may find it easier to apply these principles to your life. As an intuitive eater myself, I hope this chapter will help solidify the concepts of intuitive eating for you. These are simple principles, but they will give you a more profound understanding of what intuitive eating is truly about.

## Don't Diet

As I have mentioned frequently throughout this eBook, intuitive eating isn't a diet. Therefore, when you apply this to your life, don't think of it as starting a new diet. That way, you won't restrict yourself from eating whatever you want as long as the food you eat affects your body and mind in a positive way. If you have been an avid follower of diets, it's time to make a change. Get rid of your dieting mindset and replace it with a drive to understand your body more and learn what types of food you should eat to improve your overall health and well-being.

By far, this is my favorite principle because it helped me get rid of the bad eating habits I had acquired through the years. I have already shared how I've tried different diets and none of them worked for me. But when I learned how to eat intuitively, I immediately felt better about myself. I realized that I didn't have to restrict myself in terms of food nor did I have to feel guilty about allowing myself to eat the foods that made me feel good. By getting rid of my diet mentality, I awakened my intuition, thus, enabling me to understand my body and be kinder to myself.

When I say quash your diet mentality, I mean it. Because if you try to become an intuitive eater but in the back of your mind, you still believe that there is one diet that will help you reach your health goals, then you won't be able to truly rediscover or reawaken intuitive eating. Learn how to let your past beliefs go. It will take time and a lot of conscious effort, but in the long run, it will help you become happier, healthier, and more intuitive when it comes to food and eating. After all, if you haven't found happiness in diets, why should you allow them to hold you back?

## Respect Your Hunger Mentality

To become an intuitive eater, you should learn how to respect your hunger mentality. This means that you allow yourself to eat when you need to. But when you want to eat and you give in to this want, you won't allow yourself to feel discouraged. Needing to eat and wanting to eat are two very different things that are both part of your hunger mentality. Unfortunately, when you follow a diet, you learn how to feel bad or guilty when you allow yourself to eat just because you want to. This, in turn, makes you feel deprived and hungry all the time. But the truth is, most of the time, you're not really hungry, you just want to eat!

The trouble with depriving yourself or ignoring your hunger mentality is you are actually teaching yourself to feel bad about food and about eating. This is one of the reasons why food has become a huge stressor in our lives when it shouldn't be. Instead, you should learn how to accept your physical hunger and your desire to eat so that you can make peace with yourself. In doing this, you will come to understand your hunger mentality, and, in time, you will learn how to control it too.

Don't allow yourself to reach the point where you feel excessively hungry because you keep denying yourself nourishment. This will only lead to overeating. Make sure to always provide your body with the nourishment it needs to feel satisfied. In doing this, you may notice that you don't focus on food all the time. Since you have built a healthier relationship with food by respecting your hunger mentality, you can stop worrying about whether you are "doing things right" or not. You can focus on other things and rely on your intuition to tell you when it's time to eat and how much you should eat when you feel hungry.

## Learn How to Have Fun With Food

The longer you stick with intuitive eating, the more it becomes a positive thing for you. In the past, you might have perceived food as "the enemy" that was preventing you from leading a happier, healthier life. Because of this, you always associated food with negative emotions. But to become an intuitive eater, you must turn things around. Instead of feeling bad about food, learn how to have fun with it!

Stop resisting your urge to eat and allow yourself to feel happy when you do. You have probably noticed that when you stop yourself from eating a certain type of food, you end up feeling intensely deprived. The more you restrict yourself, the more intense these feelings become. And when you reach your breaking point, you end up giving in to your cravings which, in turn, may lead to bingeing. Then after giving in and eating too much, you start feeling guilty about what you did. This is a common cycle that creates the negativity you have when it comes to food. If this situation sounds familiar to you, it's time to make a change.

Food is a basic necessity. You need it to nourish your mind and body. Without food, you won't survive. To have fun with food, open yourself to trying new things by experimenting with different types of food, different dishes, and even different cuisines. Always look for new ways to stimulate your taste buds and make your eating habits more interesting. When you do this, you will also learn how to have more fun with food. You don't have to try doing too many things at once as you might feel overwhelmed. Instead, try to think about what type of food you have always wanted to try but never had the courage to. Or you can also think about a food that you have always restricted yourself from eating. Start with these and allow yourself to eat. Take small steps towards feeling more positive about food so you can feel inspired to have fun with it.

## Eat What You Want to Eat

When it comes to intuitive eating, you don't have to follow rules that say what you should eat and what you should avoid. In fact, you can even enjoy the indulgent foods that many tell you to avoid at all costs. Now is the time to stop thinking that some foods are "good" while others are "bad." Stop trying to play the role of "Food Police" where you only allow yourself to eat fruits and vegetables because these are good while you restrict yourself from eating cake, pasta, and bacon because these are bad. If you keep doing this to yourself, you are only hindering yourself from becoming a true intuitive eater.

It's time to give up the Food Police that always monitors what you eat and forces you to follow unreasonably restrictive rules that you have created for yourself. Silly as it may seem, this Food Police actually lives deep within your mind and whenever negative things pop into your head that are related to food and eating, you know that your own personal authority on food has come to the surface.

The good news is that you don't have to just accept the things that the Food Police tells you. Just as you would rid yourself of your diet mentality and your negative associations with food, you can also get rid of the Food Police that is preventing you from relearning intuitive eating. Consciously make an effort to quiet that relentless voice in your head that tries to control your food intake. When you want to eat something, encourage and allow yourself to eat. If it makes you feel good, continue eating that food. If it doesn't then try to find other types of food that will make you feel healthier and more satisfied. It's all about experimentation to find what works and what doesn't so you can hone your intuition.

## Know Your Limits

After you learn how to accept food and feel more positive about your eating habits, the next thing to do is know your limits. Just because you will allow yourself to eat as much as you want or as much as you think your body needs, this doesn't mean that you should allow yourself to eat over your limit all the time. If you keep allowing yourself to do this, then you might not experience all the benefits that intuitive eating has to offer. In fact, you might even experience the opposite of what you are expecting from this eating approach.

Going back to your diet habits, you would often end up overeating or bingeing when you restrict yourself. Since you don't allow yourself to eat what you want, you end up craving the foods that you want to eat the most. But when you can't control your urges anymore, then you give in, and when you do, it's usually excessive.

But as you should know by now, intuitive eating doesn't involve restriction. Since you allow yourself to eat whatever you want, whenever you want, and continue eating until you feel satisfied, then you shouldn't have any reason to eat more than you have to. Knowing your limits is an important part of intuitive eating as this is when you learn how to tune in to your body. As you eat, try to make yourself aware of how the food makes you feel and whether you are still hungry or not. When you realize that you already feel full, this is the indication that you have reached your limit. It may take some time for you to know your limits but once you do this, it means that you would have unlocked your natural intuitive instinct. This would then make it easier for you to control yourself around food without actually trying to restrict yourself while eating.

## Associate Food With Happiness

This is one of the most important principles of intuitive eating and if you can apply it to your life, you can learn how to eat intuitively. To become an intuitive eater, food should be your happy place. It should make you feel comfortable and it should never make you feel guilty no matter what. If you want to awaken your intuition and unlock your instincts, then you should trust yourself enough around food. Remember that you are trying to determine which foods will make you feel good and which foods won't. This is a process that you shouldn't rush through. Instead, you should try and enjoy the ride.

As you allow yourself to eat the things that you want to eat, you would also tune into the signals of your body as these will tell you if you should keep eating or if you should stop because you're already full. To help move this process along, try to take a moment in the middle of your meal to notice the textures and tastes of the food you are eating. Also, try to determine your hunger level to know if you have already reached your limit or if you can still continue eating.

Then try to tune into the feelings that you get from the food that you eat. If you still feel negative emotions like guilt, shame or frustration when faced with food that you previously believed you shouldn't be eating, learn how to reassure yourself. Find ways to make the experience more positive like having a mantra, consciously trying to awaken positive emotions, learning how to appreciate the food you are eating, and more. Keep practicing this until you start associating food with happiness. Not only does food nourish your body, but it should also nourish your mind and soul for the benefit of your overall well-being.

## Focus on Other Things Too

When you focus too much on food, you might find it difficult to apply intuitive eating to your life. Focusing solely on food is something that you learn by dieting. Think about it: when you are on a diet, your main focus is on the food you should eat and the food that you shouldn't eat. So, if you continue doing this, it would still be like following a diet. Intuitive eating is more than this. Intuitive eating encourages you to focus on other things so that you can let go of the frustrations and negative emotions that you have always felt when thinking about—or even eating—food.

This is especially important when you are dealing with stressful situations. We have already discussed how emotional eating works and how you can change the trend by focusing on other things. Now that you don't have to think about food all the time, you can start focusing on other things that matter to you. For instance, when faced with emotionally charged situations, you can stop yourself from using food as your solution because you have already tuned into your body. Take a moment to find out how you truly feel. If you don't feel hungry, then don't eat. Instead, find something else to do. Something that will make you feel productive or something that will help improve your situation.

Make a conscious effort to find alternative things to focus on so your world doesn't just revolve around food. If you want food to stop controlling your life, then you have to be the one to fix your relationship. Focus is a powerful thing. If you can learn how to shift your focus with a strong sense of purpose through your intuition, then you can also learn how to listen to your body while eating. This, in turn, allows you to eat more intuitively.

## Believe That Your Body is a Temple

Speaking of tuning into your body, you must always remind yourself that your body is a temple. Keep telling yourself this until you truly believe it. Until it becomes your reality. No matter what you look like, no matter how far you are from your body goals, learn how to treat your body with the respect it deserves. Accept the fact that you were born with a specific genetic blueprint. This means that no matter how hard you try, you might not achieve the body goals that you have set for yourself, especially if you have set goals that are unreasonably high.

Rather than punishing yourself for not having the "ideal body," learn how to love and accept the body that you have. As you learn how to eat intuitively, you will also learn how to connect with your body in ways that you never even considered before. But you cannot truly connect with your body if you don't learn how to respect it. Respect comes in the form of acceptance, of learning how to listen, and of truly loving your body unconditionally.

Yes, you can still try to achieve your goals but now, you may want to set more realistic goals for yourself. Go back to the list of body goals you have created and try to determine if these are realistic enough for you. If they seem impossible, you may want to change those goals. That way, you won't put too much pressure on yourself to the point that you start feeling frustrated and negative about your body. Again, this might bring you back to your diet mentality. It might push you to run back to dieting as you would awaken your belief that there is one diet that will make you "runway ready." This is one of the more difficult principles to apply to your life. But trust me when I say that it is not impossible.

Take a stand for yourself. Look in the mirror and learn to appreciate what you see. In the same way you would make food your happy place, put in a conscious effort to change your perception of your body until you learn how to accept it—curves, blemishes, scars, and all. Then if you see positive changes happening to your body because of intuitive eating, this would make you appreciate this approach even more. It will also make you love your body more which, in turn, will motivate you to continue showing respect to your body by doing everything you can to keep it healthy and strong.

## Exercise Regularly

In Chapter 2, we already covered the importance of having a regular exercise routine as part of your intuitive eating journey. Since you will allow yourself to eat whatever you want while following this approach, exercising regularly to keep fit just makes sense. Whether you exercise to achieve your body goals, or you just do it to make yourself feel better, this type of physical activity is a must to improve your overall health and well-being.

Exercise is one thing that intuitive eating has in common with diets. Typically, diets work better when you pair them with exercise. Intuitive eating also works better when you pair it with exercise because it helps you learn more about your body.

When I suggest that you exercise regularly, I don't mean that you should go to the gym every day. These days, there are so many different types of workout routines and so many ways for you to learn them. There are workout apps, online videos, and other such resources that will allow you to exercise in the comfort of your own home. Exercising is also a great way for you to become more connected to your body. As you move, try to make yourself aware of how your muscles feel, as well as, the other parts of your body. By doing this, you will also be honing your intuition as you learn what exercises make you feel good, what exercises make your body ache, and how much exercise you can do at a time. By learning all of these things, you are also learning more about your body and how it works.

## Prioritize Your Health

The final principle of intuitive eating involves all the other principles that we have discussed. As you apply all of these to your life, you would be on your way to making health your priority. Now, it's time to start thinking about what will benefit you and what may cause you harm. For instance, when it comes to choosing food, try to stay away from food that will be detrimental to your health. Just because you don't have to restrict yourself from eating certain foods, doesn't mean that you should only eat those unhealthy foods that will start taking a toll on your health.

Let me give you a concrete example of this. For instance, you love processed meat products. When you follow a certain diet, you would probably have to stop eating these meat products altogether. But when you follow the intuitive eating approach, you may allow yourself to eat these food items, especially if they make you feel good. However, you shouldn't ignore the fact that these food products contain ingredients that can be harmful to your health, especially when eaten too frequently or in large quantities. Since you must also learn how to respect your body, only feeding it with processed meat products won't nourish it well. This means that you would be ignoring the other principles of intuitive eating to give yourself permission to only eat unhealthy food.

Intuitive eating is also about learning how to balance your wants and your needs. No, you don't have to restrict yourself from eating certain types of food. But you should also think about whether the food you eat will make you healthier or not. If you rely on your intuition, you may actually discover that eating healthy will make you healthy which, in turn, can help you reach the body goals and health objectives that you have set for yourself.

# CONCLUSION: STARTING YOUR INTUITIVE EATING JOURNEY

If you're ready to improve your eating habits for the long run, then it's time to take your intuitive eating journey now. As one who has been following this approach to eating for some time now, I can confidently say that intuitive eating has taught me to be kinder to myself and it has also taught me how to listen to my body while using my intuition to guide me.

Now that you have reached the end of this eBook, you have learned all the fundamental information to help you become a true intuitive eater. After the introduction of intuitive eating, you learned the very first step you need to take for this journey—setting goals. It's important to set your own body goals and health objectives as these will determine the plan you will make for your intuitive eating journey. When it comes to setting goals and objectives, think of what you really want. That way, you can come up with goals and objectives that will really motivate you throughout your journey.

The second chapter was all about understanding your body. Since intuitive eating involves connecting with your body more intimately, you should first learn more about it. You learned how to establish an exercise routine, how to control your urge to eat, and how to adopt a more positive attitude towards your body. All of these are essential for intuitive eating as they will allow you to become more in-tune with your body. Then we moved on to emotional eating, a way of eating that most people follow to cope with their emotions. To become an intuitive eater, you must learn how to break your habit of emotional eating. Instead, you should learn how to be more aware of your hunger so that you don't end up eating too much to cope with your feelings. As part of becoming an intuitive eater, you may want to learn other coping mechanisms to make it easier for you to handle your emotions and the situations that caused them. Fortunately, Chapter 3 is full of effective tips and strategies to help you out.

In Chapter 4, we focused on your mindset, another important aspect of intuitive eating. After tuning in to your body, you should also learn how to tune into your own mind. Your mind is a powerful tool and if you learn how to use it to approach food and eating in a more positive way, you will truly learn how to eat intuitively. Finally, in the last chapter, I shared with you the 10 principles of intuitive eating. It's essential to understand these principles and apply them to your life so that intuitive eating becomes part of your life permanently.

From start to finish, you have learned all the skills and guidelines you need to tackle intuitive eating. The great thing about having this eBook is that you can always go back to it if you feel like you need to refresh your memory or awaken your motivation anytime during your intuitive eating journey. Congratulations on reaching the end of this eBook and congratulations on making the choice to become an intuitive eater. Good luck on your journey and remember to have fun with it!.

# REFERENCES

10 principles of intuitive eating. (n.d.). Retrieved from https://www.intuitiveeating.org/10-principles-of-intuitive-eating/

10 steps to positive body image. (2018). Retrieved from https://www.nationaleatingdisorders.org/learn/general-information/ten-steps

15 personal health goal examples within your reach. (2020). Retrieved from https://examples.yourdictionary.com/15-personal-health-goal-examples-within-your-reach.html

Alton, L. (2019). 7 practical tips to achieve a positive mindset. Retrieved from https://www.success.com/7-practical-tips-to-achieve-a-positive-mindset/

Barituka, A. (2017). Body types and goals. Retrieved from http://stylevitae.com/body-types-body-goals/

Bromley, W. (2018). What is the true meaning of reasonable body goals? Retrieved from https://thevarsity.ca/2018/06/27/what-is-the-true-meaning-of-reasonable-body-goals/

Cherry, K. (2019). How can positive thinking benefit your mind and body? Retrieved from https://www.verywellmind.com/benefits-of-positive-thinking-2794767

Chua, C. (2019). 12 signs of emotional eating (and why it is bad for you). Retrieved from https://personalexcellence.co/blog/signs-of-emotional-eating/

Dewe, C. (2020). 11 tips for maintaining a positive attitude. Retrieved from https://www.lifehack.org/articles/communication/11-tips-for-maintaining-your-positive-attitude.html

Giblin, C. (2020). The 10 most important fitness goals. Retrieved from https://www.mensjournal.com/health-fitness/the-10-most-important-fitness-goals/

Glasofer, D. R. (2020). How to curb emotional eating. Retrieved from https://www.verywellmind.com/eating-in-response-to-emotion-4001635

Godoy, M. (2019). Trust your gut: A beginner's guide to intuitive eating. Retrieved from https://www.npr.org/2019/05/23/726236988/trust-your-gut-a-beginners-guide-to-intuitive-eating

Gross, A. (2019). How intuitive eating can change your mindset about dieting for good - The Winchester Institute: Dublin Ohio. Retrieved from https://www.thewinchesterinstitute.com/austens-blog/2019/1/25/how-intuitive-eating-can-change-your-mindset-about-dieting-for-good-nbsp

Haas, S. B. (2010). 5 reasons why you can't control your eating. Retrieved from https://www.psychologytoday.com/us/blog/prescriptions-life/201008/5-reasons-why-you-cant-control-your-eating

Hartley, R. (2018). How to cope with negative emotions, with or without food. Retrieved from https://www.rachaelhartleynutrition.com/blog/how-to-cope-with-negative-emotions-with-or-without-food

Hartley, R. (2019). How to reframe diet mentality thoughts in intuitive eating. Retrieved from https://www.rachaelhartleynutrition.com/blog/how-to-reframe-thoughts-in-intuitive-eating

Health guides: Health is a state of mind and body. (2017). Retrieved from https://familydoctor.org/health-guides-health-state-mind-body/

Heaney, K. (2019). What does intuitive eating even mean? Retrieved from https://www.thecut.com/2019/06/what-is-intuitive-eating-a-guide-to-intuitive-eating.html

Holbrook, S. (2019). Intuitive eating is a happier and healthier way to eat-here's how to begin. Retrieved from https://www.realsimple.com/health/nutrition-diet/healthy-eating/intuitive-eating

How to build an exercise plan. (2020). Retrieved from https://www.helpguide.org/harvard/whats-the-best-exercise-plan-for-me.htm

Jennings, K.-A. (2019). A quick guide to intuitive eating. Retrieved from https://www.healthline.com/nutrition/quick-guide-intuitive-eating

Kromberg, J. (2013). Emotional eating? 5 reasons you can't stop. Retrieved from https://www.psychologytoday.com/us/blog/inside-out/201309/emotional-eating-5-reasons-you-can-t-stop

Laliberte, M. (2019). 7 ways to stop your strongest food cravings. Retrieved from https://www.thehealthy.com/weight-loss/stop-food-cravings/

Leal, D. (2020). Improve your health, mind, and body with intuitive eating. Retrieved from https://www.verywellfit.com/overview-of-intuitive-eating-4178361

MacMillan, A. (2018). What is intuitive eating? A nutritionist weighs in on this popular anti-diet. Retrieved from https://www.health.com/nutrition/intuitive-eating

Marcin, A. (2018). Emotional eating: Why it happens and how to stop it. Retrieved from https://www.healthline.com/health/emotional-eating#1

McAulay, L. (2017). 8 steps to self-care: How to love your body. Retrieved from https://www.healthline.com/health/8-ways-to-embrace-self-love-and-thank-your-body#1

McCoy, J. (2019). 11 tips to set realistic fitness goals you'll actually achieve, according to top trainers. Retrieved from https://www.self.com/story/how-to-set-realistic-fitness-goals

Miller, S. G. (2016). The science of hunger: How to control it and fight cravings. Retrieved from https://www.livescience.com/54248-controlling-your-hunger.html#longterm

Mull, A. (2019). The latest diet trend is not dieting. Retrieved from https://www.theatlantic.com/health/archive/2019/02/intuitive-eating/583357/

Neithercott, T. (2012). 11 steps to setting your health goals. Retrieved from http://www.diabetesforecast.org/2012/dec/11-steps-to-setting-your-health-goals.html

Patton, C. (2019). The importance of a positive mindset on success. Retrieved from https://thriveglobal.com/stories/the-importance-of-a-positive-mindset-on-success/

Physical activity – setting yourself goals. (2015). Retrieved from https://www.betterhealth.vic.gov.au/health/HealthyLiving/physical-activity-setting-yourself-goals

Rettner, R. (2016). How to start an exercise routine and stick to it. Retrieved from https://www.livescience.com/54805-best-way-to-start-exercising.html

Rumsey, A. (2018). How to deal with emotional eating and stress eating - Intuitive eating. Retrieved from https://alissarumsey.com/intuitive-eating/how-to-deal-with-emotional-eating/

Rumsey, A. (2019). What Is intuitive eating and how is it different from mindful eating? Retrieved from https://alissarumsey.com/intuitive-eating/what-is-intuitive-eating/

Rumsey, A. (2019). 24 intuitive eating benefits: Alissa Rumsey nutrition. Retrieved from https://alissarumsey.com/intuitive-eating/intuitive-eating-benefits/

Rumsey, A. (2019). How to shift your mindset to move towards intuitive eating. Retrieved from https://alissarumsey.com/intuitive-eating/how-to-shift-your-mindset-move-towards-intuitive-eating/

Smith, M., Segal, J., & Segal, R. (2019). Emotional eating. Retrieved from https://www.helpguide.org/articles/diets/emotional-eating.htm

The 10 principles of intuitive eating. (n.d.). Retrieved from https://eatuitive.com/blog/the-10-principles-of-intuitive-eating/

Tips to stop emotional eating. (2018). Retrieved from https://www.mayoclinic.org/healthy-lifestyle/weight-loss/in-depth/weight-loss/art-20047342

Tracy, B. (2015). Personal health and fitness through goal setting. Retrieved from https://www.briantracy.com/blog/personal-success/personal-health-and-fitness-through-goal-setting-personal-goals-set-goals/

www.ingramcontent.com/pod-product-compliance
Lightning Source LLC
Chambersburg PA
CBHW062201100526
44589CB00014B/1906